The Definitive Mediterranean Diet Cooking Guide

Easy and Affordable Fish and Meat Recipes for Incredibly Healthy Meal

Camila Lester

Table of contents

Mediterranean Pressure Pot Chicken And Potatoes

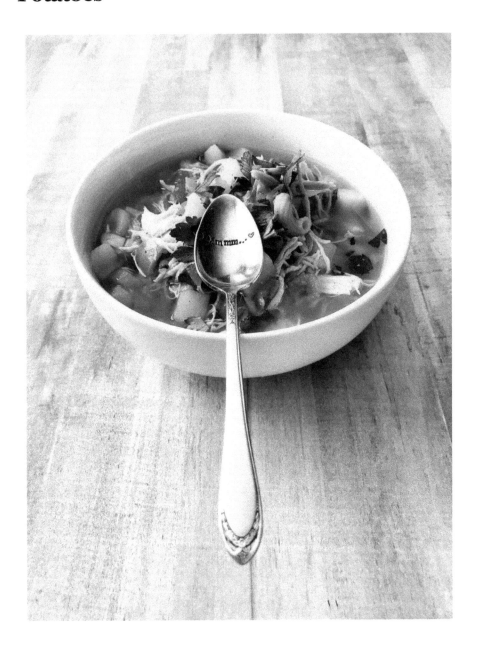

Difficulty Level: 2/5

Preparation time: 5 minutes

Cooking time: 14 Minutes

Servings: 6

Ingredients:

2 tablespoons of olive oil

½ teaspoon of ground pimento

1 teaspoon of smoked paprika

6 chicken thighs, bone in and skin on

1 cup of chicken broth

1 teaspoon of garlic puree

juice from 1 lemon

2 tablespoons of honey

1 pound of potatoes, cut in half

1 teaspoon of fresh oregano

Directions:

In a bowl, combine 1 tablespoon of olive oil with salt, smoked paprika and pimento.

Add in the chicken thighs and coat well with the sauce.

Take the other tablespoon of olive oil in the Pressure Pot using the saute setting. Add the chicken thighs and brown on both sides, about 6 minutes.

Turn the Pressure Pot off. Remove any excess oil before going further.

Pour in chicken broth.

Add in remaining ingredients, put on the lid and lock. Set the valve to the sealing position.

Set the Pressure Pot to pressure cook, high pressure for 8 minutes.

Allow for 5 minutes of natural pressure release, then perform quick pressure release for remaining.

Nutrition: (Per serving)

Calories: 273

Protein: 24 grams

Total Fat: 10 grams

Carbohydrates: 21 grams

Pressure Pot Moroccan Chicken

Difficulty Level: 2/5

Preparation time: 5 minutes

Cooking time: 25 minutes

Servings: 4

Ingredients:

1 teaspoon paprika

1 teaspoon turmeric

1 teaspoon ground cumin

½ teaspoon salt

¼ teaspoon black pepper

3 tablespoons olive oil

1 ½ pounds chicken thighs, boneless and skinless

1 ½ cups chicken broth

2 garlic cloves, minced

½ cup onions, diced

1 teaspoon ginger, minced

¾ cup quinoa, uncooked

1 can chickpeas, drained

½ cup dried cherries

chopped cilantro leaves

Directions:

Mix together paprika, turmeric, cumin, salt, and pepper in a small bowl.

Coat the chicken thighs with spice rub. Set aside.

Add 2 tablespoons of olive oil to the bottom of the Pressure Pot.

Select sauté mode.

Add chicken to the Pressure Pot and cook both sides until slightly brown. Remove from the Pressure Pot and set aside on a plate.

Add another tablespoon of olive oil to the bottom of the pot.

Add garlic, onions, and ginger, then sauté for 2 minutes while stirring slowly.

Add quinoa, dried cherries, chickpeas, chicken broth, and the browned chicken.

Close the lid and seal.

Press poultry and set for 10 minutes.

At the end of the 10 minutes, use tongs to turn the knob for quick release of pressure carefully.

Once the pressure is released, carefully open the lid.

Check the chicken and make sure it is 165 degrees F before serving.

Serve on a plate with cilantro garnish.

Energy Value Per Serving:

Calories: 194.2

Protein: 28.1 grams

Total Fat: 6.7 grams

Carbohydrates: 5.3 grams

Mediterranean Pressure Pot Shredded Beef

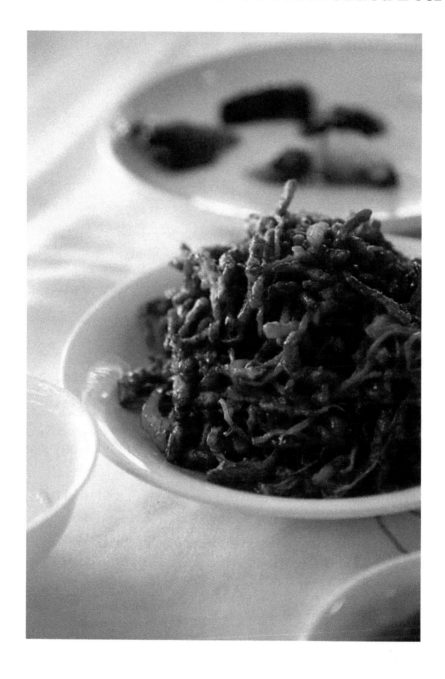

Difficulty Level: 2/5

Preparation time: 5 minutes

Cooking time: 25 minutes

Servings: 8

Ingredients:

2 pounds Chuck beef roast

1 teaspoon salt

1 cup white onion, chopped

¾ cup carrots, chopped

¾ cup yellow bell pepper, chopped

14.5 ounce can of fire-roasted tomatoes

2 tablespoons red wine vinegar

1 tablespoon garlic, minced

1 tablespoon Italian seasoning blend

1/2 tablespoon dried red pepper flakes

Directions:

Cut the beef roast into small chunks, and trim away any excess fat. Season with salt.

Place the small beef cubes into the Pressure Pot and then top with onions, carrots, and yellow bell peppers.

Open the can of fire-roasted tomatoes and stir in the vinegar, garlic, Italian dressing, and red pepper flakes. Pour mixture over the beef in the Pressure Pot.

Secure the lid and set the vent to sealed. Set for 20 minutes on the high-pressure setting.

When the timer goes off, quick release to remove pressure, remove lid carefully, and let stand for 5-10 minutes.

Use a large fork to shred beef into bite-sized pieces and then serve.

Energy Value Per Serving:

Calories: 190.2

Protein: 23.5 grams

Total Fat: 6.3 grams

Carbohydrates: 8.9 grams

Pressure Pot Orzo With Shrimp, Tomatoes, And Feta

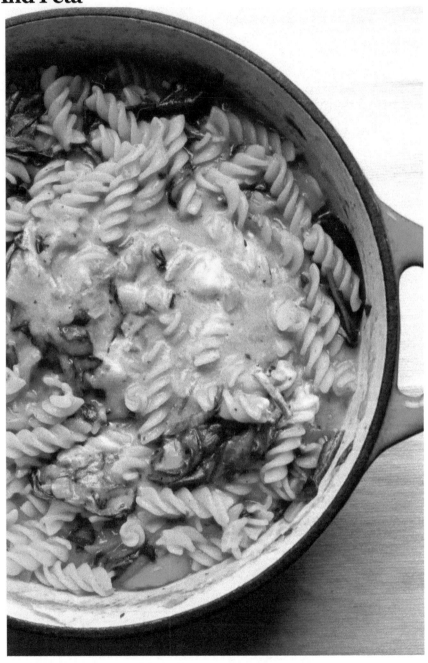

Difficulty Level: 2/5

Preparation time: 5 minutes

Cooking time: 28 Minutes

Servings: 4

Ingredients:

1 tablespoon olive oil

1 medium onion, diced

2 cloves garlic, minced

two, 14-ounce cans diced tomatoes

2 tablespoons fresh parsley

2 tablespoons fresh dill

1-¼ pounds medium shrimp, peeled and deveined

¼ teaspoon salt

¼ teaspoon freshly ground black pepper

⅔ cup of feta cheese, crumbled

1-¼ cups chicken stock

¾ cup orzo

Directions:

Set your Pressure Pot to sauté. Then add the olive oil, onion, and garlic. Cook, stirring until softened and translucent, which takes about 3 minutes. Deglaze with a splash of water to prevent sticking.

Next, add the tomatoes and chicken stock and bring to a boil, and stir.

Add the orzo, dill, and parsley and mix well.

Add shrimp and season with salt and pepper and add feta cheese.

Set Pressure Pot on manual high pressure for 3 minutes.

After 3 minutes, press the quick release to avoid overcooking the shrimp and orzo. Serve.

Energy Value Per Serving:

Calories: 395

Protein: 38 grams

Total Fat: 11 grams

Carbohydrates: 33 grams

Pressure Pot Mediterranean Chicken Wings
Difficulty Level: 2/5

Preparation time: 5 minutes

Cooking time: 13 minutes

Servings: 2

Ingredients:

1 pound of chicken wings

1 tablespoon garlic puree

3 tablespoons coconut oil

6 tablespoons white wine

1 tablespoon chicken seasoning

3 tablespoons tarragon

1 tablespoon oregano

1 tablespoon basil

salt and pepper to taste

1 cup of water

Directions:

Split the marinade ingredients between two foil sheets.

Split the chicken wings between the two parcels and rub well into the mixture. Seal each package up and shake so everything has a good coating.

Add one cup of water to your Pressure Pot and place the steaming shelf on top.

Place chicken wing packets on top of the steaming shelf.

Place the lid on your Pressure Pot and set the valve to sealing, then press manual button for 10 minutes.

Ready to serve in foil packets.

Energy Value Per Serving:

Calories: 545

Protein: 26 grams

Total Fat: 42 grams

Carbohydrates: 8 grams

Pressure Pot Lemon Pepper Salmon

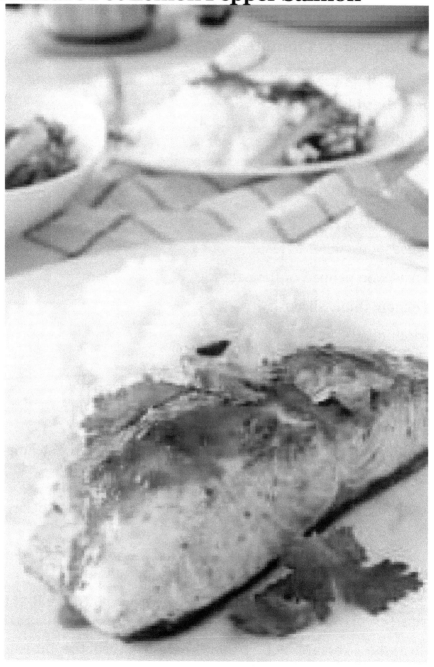

Difficulty Level: 2/5

Preparation time: 5 minutes

Cooking time: 15 minutes

Servings: 4

Ingredients:

¾ cup of water

a few sprigs parsley, tarragon, and basil

1 pound salmon filet, skin on

3 teaspoons ghee butter

¼ teaspoon salt, or to taste

½ teaspoon pepper, or to taste

½ lemon, thinly sliced

1 zucchini

1 red bell pepper

1 carrot

Directions:

Put the water and herbs in the Pressure Pot and then the steamer.

Place the salmon with the skin side down on the rack.

Drizzle on some ghee, season with salt and pepper for desired taste, and cover with lemon slices.

Close the Pressure Pot and make sure the vent is turned to "sealing." Press the steam button and set for 3 minutes.

While the salmon is cooking, cut all the veggies into small, thin strips.

When the Pressure Pot is done, quick release the pressure carefully. After pressure is released, press keep warm.

Open the lid using mitts and carefully remove the rack with the salmon on it and set on a plate.

Discard the herbs. Add the veggies and put the lid back on, then press the sauté setting. Let the veggies cook for 1-2 minutes.

Serve veggies with salmon and add remaining teaspoon of ghee to the pot.

Energy Value Per Serving:

Calories: 296

Protein: 31 grams

Total Fat: 15 grams

Carbohydrates: 8 grams

Chicken & Vegetable Wraps

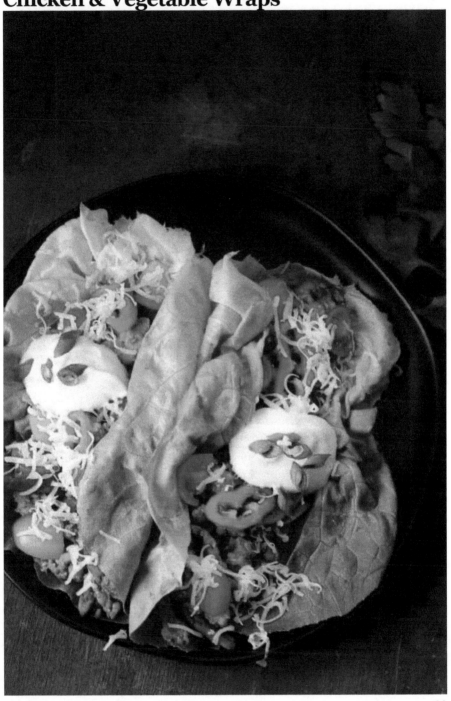

Difficulty Level: 1/5

Preparation time: 15 minutes

Cooking time: 0 min.

Servings: 4

Ingredients:

¼ cup Plain Greek Yogurt

2 cups Chicken, cooked and chopped

½ Red Bell Pepper, diced

½ English Cucumber, diced

½ cup Carrot, shredded

1 Scallion, chopped

½ tsp Fresh Thyme, chopped

1 Tbsp Fresh Lemon Juice

4 Multigrain Tortillas

Directions:

In a large bowl, mix cucumber, red bell pepper, chicken, scallion, carrot, lemon juice, thyme, yogurt, sea salt and pepper.

Spoon a quarter of this mixture into each tortilla, folding it over to make a pocket.

Repeat with remaining ingredients.

Nutrition:

Calories: 278

Protein: 27 Grams

Fat: 7 Grams

Carbs: 28 Grams

Kale Chicken Soup

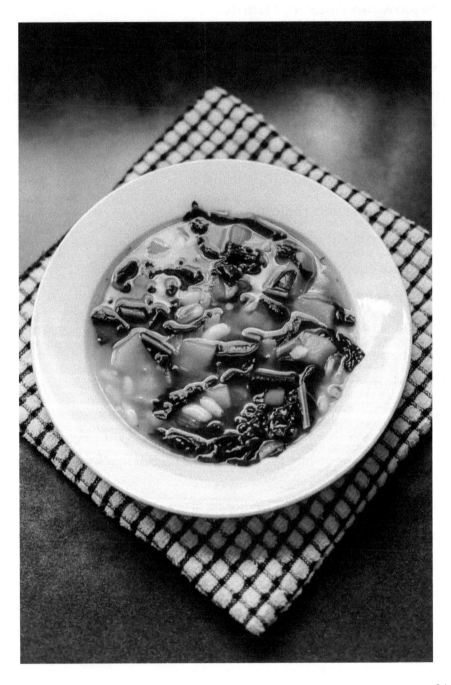

Difficulty Level: 2/5

Preparation time: 5 minutes

Cooking time: 20 min.

Servings: 2

Ingredients:

1½ Tbsp Olive Oil

11½ Cups Kale, chopped

½ cup Carrot, minced

1 Cloves Garlic, minced

4 Cups Chicken Broth, low sodium

¾ cup Patina Pasta, uncooked

1 Cups Chicken, cooked & shredded

1½ Tbsp Parmesan Cheese, grated

Directions:

In a stock pot, preheat olive oil and cooking for 30 seconds. Stir often, add carrot and kale. Cook 5 minutes, continuously stirring.

Add broth, pepper, salt turning the heat to high. Bring it to a boil before adding in pasta.

Cook for ten minutes on medium heat. Pasta should be cooked, stir occasionally so it doesn't stick to the bottom.

Add chicken meat and cook more 2 minutes.

Ladle the soup and serve topped with cheese.

Nutrition:

Calories: 187

Protein: 15 Grams

Fat: 5 Grams

Carbs: 16 Grams

Parmesan Chicken Wraps

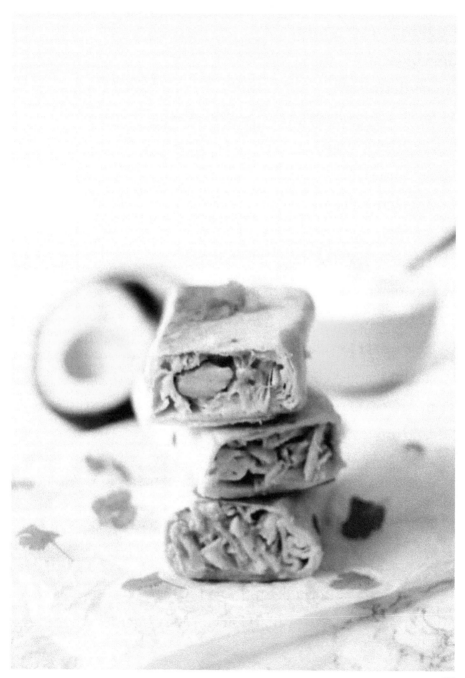

Difficulty Level: 2/5

Preparation time: 25 minutes

Cooking time: 5 min.

Servings: 2

Ingredients:

½ Lb. Chicken breasts, boneless & skinless

2/3 cup whole wheat panko bread crumbs

½ egg, large

¼ cup buttermilk

½ cup parmesan cheese, grated

¾ tsp garlic powder, divided

½ cup tomatoes, salt free & crushed

½ tsp oregano

2 whole wheat tortilla, 8 inches each

½ cup mozzarella cheese, fresh & sliced

1 cup flat leaf parsley, loosely packed, fresh & chopped

Directions:

Pre heat oven to 425 ° F. Cover the baking sheet with foil. Put the wire rack on top of it. Coat wire rack in nonstick spray, set it to the side.

Put the chicken breasts in a zipper top plastic bag. Pound chicken so that it's ¼ inch thick with a rolling pin or meat mallet. Slice it into 2 portions.

Whisk egg and buttermilk together in shallow bowl.

Mix parmesan, panko crumbs and garlic powder together in the another shallow bowl.

Dip chicken into the egg mixture and then the crumb mixture. Press the crumbs into the chicken, and then place them on the wire rack.

Bake for fifteen to eighteen minutes, and then slice diagonally

In a microwave safe bowl, mix tomatoes, remaining garlic powder and oregano together. Microwave for 1 minute and set it to the side.

Wrap tortillas with a damp paper towel and then microwave for thirty seconds.

Assemble with chicken and cheese, and then spread warm tomato sauce over each one.

Serve warm.

Nutrition:

Calories: 174

Protein: 18 Grams

Fat: 4 Grams

Carbs: 16 Grams

Cod & Green Bean Dinner

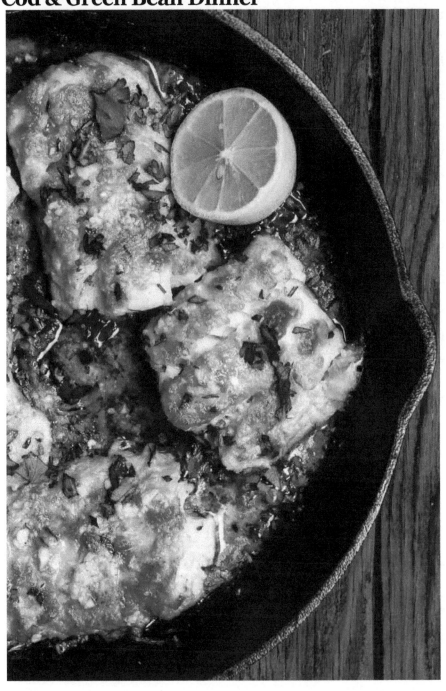

Difficulty Level: 2/5

Preparation time: 10 minutes

Cooking time: 10 min.

Serves: 2

Ingredients:

1 Tbsp Olive Oil

½ Tbsp Balsamic Vinegar

2 Cod Fillets, 4 oz. Each

1 ½ Cups Green Beans

½ Pint Cherry Grapes

Directions:

Heat oven to 390° F, and get out two rimmed baking sheets. Coat them with nonstick cooking spray.

Whisk vinegar and oil together in the bowl before setting it to the side.

Place two pieces of fish on each baking sheet.

Get out a bowl and combine tomatoes and beans.

Pour the oil and vinegar over it, and toss to coat.

Pour half of the green bean mixture over the fish on one baking sheet and the remaining fish and green beans on the other.

Turn the fish over, and coat it with the oil mixture.

Bake for five to eight minutes.

Nutrition:

Calories: 440

Protein: 14 Grams

Fat: 22 Grams

Carbs: 48 Grams

Easy Grilled Catfish

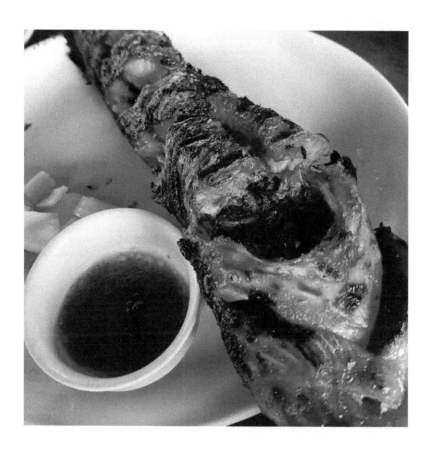

Difficulty Level: 2/5

Preparation time: 10 minutes

Cooking time: 15 min.

Servings: 4

Ingredients:

2 Lemons

2 Catfish Fillets, 4 oz. Each

½ Tbsp Olive Oil

Sea Salt & Black Pepper to Taste

Directions:

Pat fish dry with paper towels, and allow to stand at room temperature for ten minutes.

Coat the grill with cooking spray, and preheat it to 375° F.

Cut one of the lemons in half, and then set half of it aside.

Slice one half into ¼ inch slices.

Get out a bowl and squeeze a tablespoon of juice from the reserved half.

Mix lemon juice and oil in a bowl, and brush fish with it.

Season with salt and pepper.

Place the lemon slices on the grill, and place fish fillets on each one.

Turn the fish halfway through.

 Serve with lemon.

Nutrition:

Calories: 323

Protein: 56 Grams

Fat: 10 Grams

Carbs: 0 Grams

Garlic & Orange Shrimp

Difficulty Level: 2/5

Preparation time: 10 minutes

Cooking time: 10 min

Servings: 2

Ingredients:

3 Cloves Garlic, minced

Sea Salt & Black Pepper to taste

2 ½ oz. Shrimp, Fresh & Raw, de-shelled & tails removed

½ Tbsp Thyme, fresh & chopped

½ Tbsp Rosemary, fresh & chopped

1½ Tbsp Olive Oil, divided

½ Orange, large

Directions:

Zest orange. In a zippertop back, combine zest with 1 Tbsp of oil and rosemary. Add in garlic, pepper, salt and thyme.

Add in shrimp, and seal. Massage the seasoning into the shrimp and set aside.

Heat a grill, and then brush the remaining oil onto shrimp.

Cook for 4-6 minutes in a grill pan, and flip halfway through.

Transfer to a serving bowl, and then chop orange.

Serve with shrimp.

Nutrition:

Calories: 327

Protein: 31 Grams

Fat: 5 Grams

Carbs: 40 Grams

Kale & Tuna Bowl

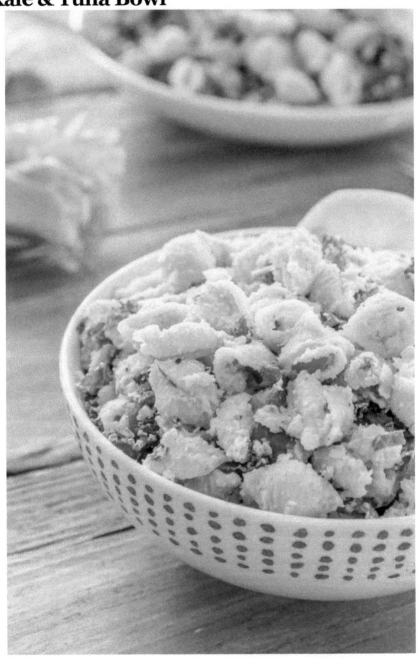

Difficulty Level: 2/5

Preparation time: 5 minutes

Cooking time: 15 min.

Serves: 2

Ingredients:

½ lb. Kale, Chopped

1½ Tbsp Olive Oil

1 oz. Olives, Canned & Drained

1½Cloves Garlic, Minced

½ cup Onion, Chopped

¼ cup Capers

¼ Tsp Crushed Red Pepper

1 Tsps Sugar

1 Cans Tuna in Olive Oil, Undrained & 6 oz. Each1

7 Ounce Can Cannellini Beans, Drained & Rinsed

½ a dash of salt

½ a dash of pepper

Directions:

Fill a large stockpot three quarters full of water.

Bring it to a boil and cook kale for 2 minutes. Drain in colander before setting aside.

Place empty pot over medium heat, and then add in oil.

Add in onion, and cook for 4 minutes. Stir often and cook garlic for a minute more.

Stir often, and then add the olives, crushed red pepper, capers, and cook for 1 minute. Stir often, and add kale and sugar in. Stir well, and cook for 8 minutes while covered.

Remove from heat, and mix in tuna, pepper, salt, and beans.

Serve warm.

Nutrition:

Calories: 265

Protein: 16 Grams

Fat: 12 Grams

Carbs: 26 Grams

Salmon & Avocado Salad

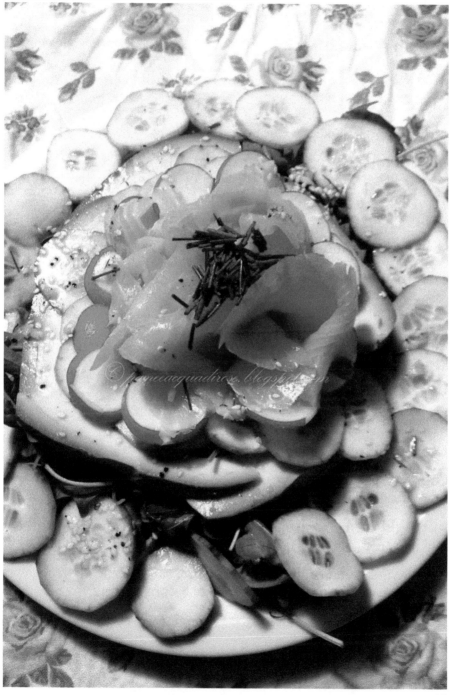

Difficulty Level: 2/5

Preparation time: 25-30 minutes

Cooking time: 0 min.

Servings: 2

Ingredients:

1 lb. Salmon, Cooked & Chopped

1 lb. Shrimp, Cooked & Chopped

½ cup Avocado, Chopped

4 cups green such as spinach or spring mix

½ cup Mayonnaise

2 Tbsp Lime Juice, Fresh

1 Clove Garlic

½ cup Sour Cream

Sea Salt & Black Pepper to Taste

½ Red Onion, Minced

½ cup Cucumber, Chopped

Directions:

Combine garlic, salt, pepper, onion, mayonnaise, sour cream and lime juice in the bowl,

In the different bowl mix together salmon, shrimp, cucumber, and avocado.

Add the mayonnaise mixture to shrimp, salmon and then allow it to sit for twenty minutes in the fridge before serving.

Nutrition:

Calories: 309

Protein: 28 Grams

Fat: 13 Grams

Carbs: 18 Grams

Salmon Salad Wraps

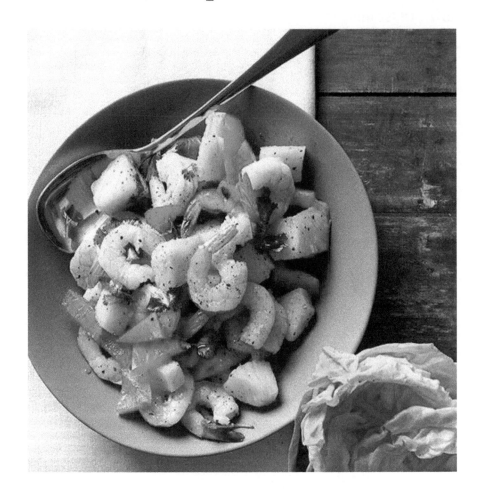

Difficulty Level: 2/5

Preparation time: 20 minutes

Cooking time: 0 min.

Servings: 2

Ingredients:

½ lb. Salmon Fillet, cooked & flaked

½ cup Carrots, diced

½ cup Celery, diced

1 Tbsp Red Onion, diced

1Tbsp Dill, fresh & diced

1 Tbsp Capers

½ Tbsp Aged Balsamic Vinegar

½ Tbsp Olive Oil

½ a dash of salt

½ a dash of pepper

2 Whole Wheat Flatbread Wraps

Directions:

Mix carrots, dill, celery, salmon, red onions, oil, vinegar, pepper, capers and salt together in the bowl.

Divide between flatbread, and fold up to serve.

Nutrition:

Calories: 336

Protein: 32 Grams

Fat: 16 Grams

Carbs: 23 Grams

Scallops In Citrus Sauce

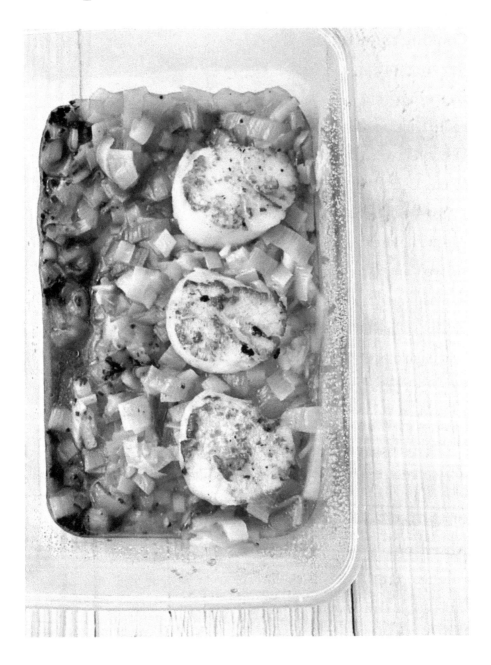

Difficulty Level: 2/5

Preparation time: 10 minutes

Cooking time: 10 min.

Servings: 2

Ingredients:

2 tsp olive oil

½ shallot, minced

10 sea scallops, cleaned

½ tsp lime zest

½ tbsp lemon zest

2 tsp orange zest

½ tbsp fresh basil, chopped

½ cup fresh orange juice

½ tbsp fresh lemon juice

½ tbsp raw honey

½ tbsp plain Greek yogurt

½ tsp fine sea salt

1 tbsp Provencal herbs

Directions:

In large skillet, pour olive oil and heat over medium-high heat.

Add in minced shallot and sauté for 1 minute.

Add shallots and cook until soft.

In cold water, rinse scallops and pat dry with towel. In the skillet, pour 1 tablespoon of olive oil, sprinkle with salt and Provencal herbs.

Add scallops in and sear for 2 minutes.

Turn once during this time. They should be tender.

Push scallops to the edge of the skillet, stirring in three zests, basil, lemon juice, and orange juice.

It will boil and the scallops with absorb the flavorful liquid.

Let the scallops stay in the pan for exactly 2 minutes with the juice and turn off the heat.

Cook in saucepan for 2 minutes on medium heat.

Coat scallops in sauce before serving warm.

Nutrition:

Calories: 207

Protein: 26 Grams

Fat: 4 Grams

Carbs: 17 Grams

Shrimp Salad

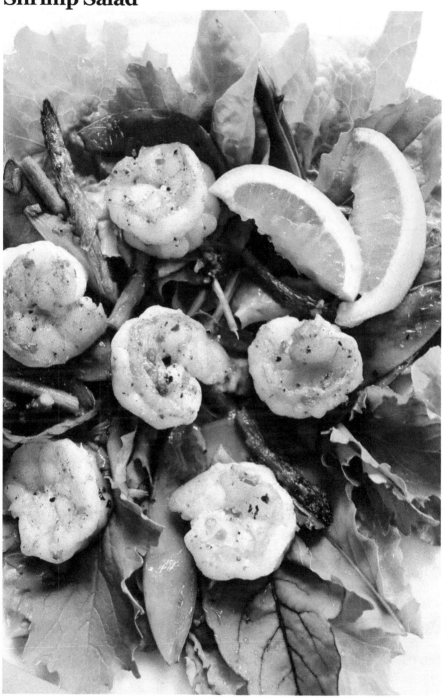

Difficulty Level: 2/5

Preparation time: 10 minutes

Cooking time: 0 min.

Servings: 2

Ingredients:

1 lbs. Shrimp, cleaned & cooked

1 celery stalks, fresh

½ onion

1 green onions

2 eggs, boiled

1½ potatoes, cooked

1½ tbsp mayonnaise

½ a dash of salt

½ a dash of black pepper

Directions:

Slice potatoes and chop celery.

Slice eggs and season.

Mix everything together.

Put shrimp over the eggs, and then serve with onions.

Nutrition:

Calories: 360

Protein: 31 Grams

Fat: 14 Grams

Carbs: 32 Grams

Trout & Greens
Difficulty Level: 2/5

Preparation time: 30 minutes

Cooking time: 0 min.

Servings: 2

Ingredients:

½ tsp Olive Oil (plus extra for greasing)

1 cup Swiss Chard, chopped

1 cup Kale, chopped

¼ Sweet Onion, thinly-sliced

1 5-oz Trout Fillet, skin on

¼ Lemon, zested

Pinch of Fine Salt

Pinch of Black Pepper

½ a bunch of parsley

Pinch of Black Pepper

Directions:

Preheat oven to 395 degrees.

Defrost trout if frozen, rinse, cut fins, head and tail.

Dry with paper towels.

Slice lemons and halve each slice.

Finely chop parsley.

Rub the fish inside and out with ground black pepper.

Fill the trout abdomen with greens.

Make diagonal cuts on one side of the trout.

Insert a half cup of lemon into each of them.

Sprinkle fish with lemon juice and olive oil.

Grease a 9x13 inch baking dish using olive oil.

Lay out on a baking dish Swiss chard, kale, and onion.

Put the fish on top of vegetables.

Make sure the skin side is up.

Serve with lemon zest after seasoning.

Nutrition:

Calories: 120

Protein: 17 Grams

Fat: 5 Grams

Carbs: 0 Grams

Bean And Tuna Salad

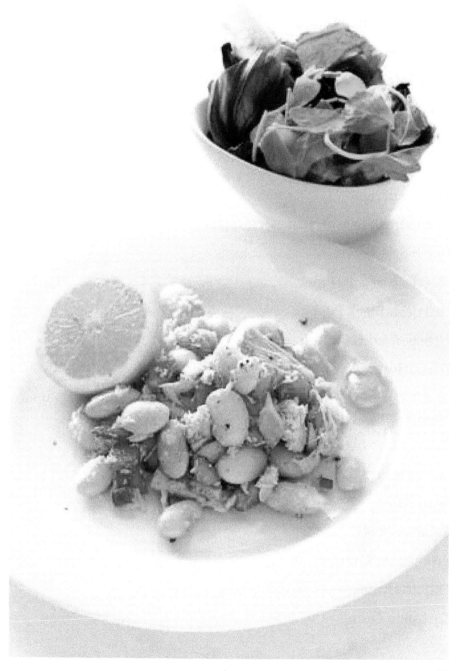

Difficulty Level: 2/5

Preparation time: 15 minutes

Cooking time: 0 min

Servings: 2

Ingredients:

½ can white beans, rinsed and drained

½ cup cooked tuna, broken into chunks

½ red onion, chopped

½ juice of lemon

½ cup fresh parsley leaves, chopped

½ tsp dried mint

½ a dash of salt, Fine

½ a dash Black Pepper

1 Tbsp of extra virgin olive oil

Directions:

In a deep bowl, toss to combine tuna chunks, beans, parsley, onions, mint, olive oil, lemon juice.

Season with black pepper, salt.

Serve chilled.

Nutrition:

Calories: 335

Protein: 20 Grams

Fat: 20 Grams

Carbs: 22 Grams

Tuna Sandwiches

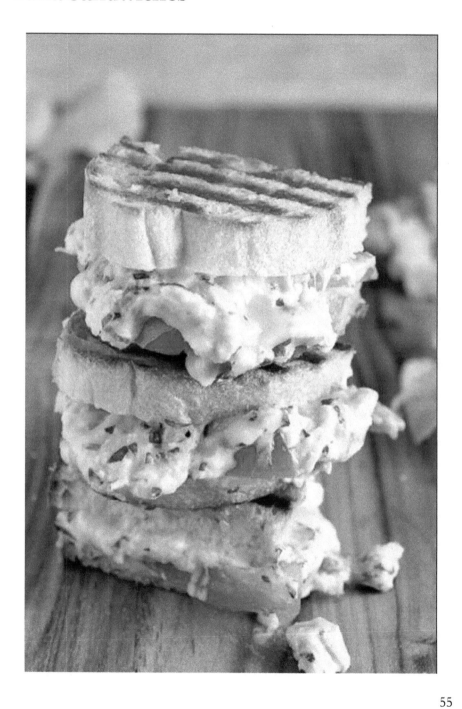

Difficulty Level: 2/5

Preparation time: 30 minutes

Cooking time: 0 min.

Servings: 4

Ingredients:

1½Tbsp Lemon Juice, fresh

1 Tbsp Olive Oil

Sea Salt & Black Pepper to taste

½ Clove Garlic, minced

2½ oz. Canned Tuna, drained

Ounce Canned Olives, sliced

½ cup Fennel, fresh & chopped

4 Slices Whole Grain Bread

Directions:

In a bowl, whisk lemon juice, garlic, pepper and oil before adding in fennel, olive sand tuna.

Use a fork to separate it into chunks before mixing everything together.

Divide between four slices of bread.

Serve it.

Nutrition:

Calories: 332

Protein: 29 Grams

Fat: 12 Grams

Carbs: 27 Grams

Tuna With Lettuce And Chickpeas
Difficulty Level: 2/5

Preparation time: 25 minutes

Cooking time: 0 min

Servings: 2

Ingredients:

½ head green lettuce, washed cut in thin strips

½ cup chopped watercress

½ cucumber, peeled and chopped

½ tomato, diced

½ can tuna, drained and broken into small chunks

¼ cup chickpeas, from a can

3-4 radishes, sliced

1½-2 spring onions, chopped

juice of half lemon

1½- Tbsp extra-virgin olive oil

Directions:

Mix green lettuce, watercress, cucumber, tomato, radishes, spring onion in a large bowl.

Add to the vegetables the tuna and the chickpeas.

Toss over with lemon juice, oil and salt to taste.

Nutrition:

Calories: 290

Protein: 14 Grams

Fat: 22 Grams

Carbs: 8 Grams

Chicken with Salsa & Cilantro

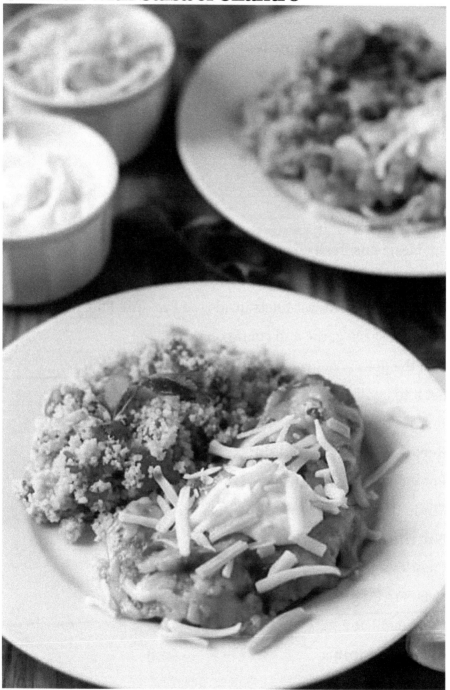

Difficulty Level: 2/5

Preparation time: 10 minutes

Cooking time: 15 minutes

Servings: 6

Ingredients:

1 ½ lb. chicken breast fillets

2 cups salsa verde

1 teaspoon garlic, minced

1 teaspoon cumin

2 tablespoons fresh cilantro, chopped

Directions:

Put the chicken breast fillets inside the Pressure Pot.

Pour the salsa, garlic and cumin on top.

Seal the pot.

Set it to poultry.

Release the pressure quickly.

Remove the chicken and shred.

Put it back to the pot.

Stir in the cilantro.

Nutrition: (Per serving)

Calories 238

Total Fat 8.7g

Saturated Fat 2.3g

Cholesterol 101mg

Sodium 558mg

Total Carbohydrate 3.8g

Dietary Fiber 0.4g

Total Sugars 1.2g

Protein 34g

Potassium 285mg

Cacciatore Black Olive Chicken

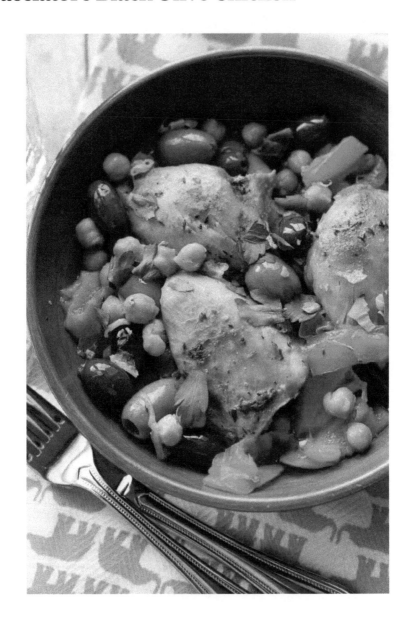

Difficulty Level: 2/5

Preparation time: 10 minutes

Cooking time: 15 minutes

Servings: 4-6

Ingredients

6–8 bone-in chicken drumsticks or mixed drumsticks and thighs

1 cup chicken stock

1 bay leaf

½ cup black olives, pitted

1 medium yellow onion, roughly chopped

1 teaspoon dried oregano

1 teaspoon garlic powder

1 (28-ounce) can stewed tomato puree

Directions

Open the top lid of your Pressure Pot.

Add the stock, bay leaf and salt; stir to combine with a wooden spatula.

Add the chicken, tomato puree, onion, garlic powder and oregano; stir again.

Close the lid and make sure that the valve is sealed properly.

Press MANUAL and set timer to 15 minutes.

The Pressure Pot will start building pressure; allow the mixture to cook for the set time.

When the timer reads zero, press NPR for natural pressure release. It will take 8–10 minutes to release the pressure.

Open the lid and remove the bay leaf.

Serve warm with the black olives on top.

Nutrition (per serving)

Calories 309,

Fat 16.5 g,

Carbs 9 g,

Protein 30.5 g,

Sodium 833 mg

Mustard Green Chicken

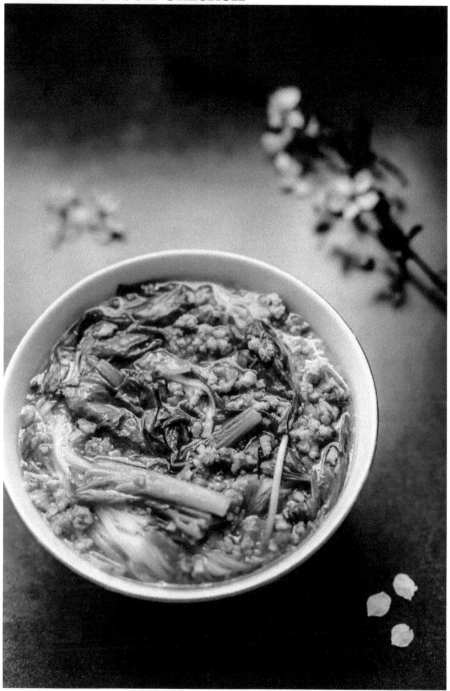

Difficulty Level: 2/5

Preparation time 10 minutes

Cooking time 15 minutes

Servings: 4

Ingredients

1 bunch mustard greens, washed and chopped

Juice of 1 lemon

⅓ cup extra-virgin olive oil

4–5 boneless, skinless chicken thighs

3 cloves garlic, minced

1 cup white wine

1 teaspoon Dijon mustard

1 teaspoon honey

½ cup cherry tomatoes

½ cup green olives, pitted

Salt and pepper to taste

Directions

Open the top lid of your Pressure Pot.

Add the mustard greens and then add the chicken thighs on top; season to taste with salt and pepper.

Top with the garlic, tomatoes, olives, mustard and honey followed by the lemon juice, olive oil and wine.

Close the lid and make sure that the valve is sealed properly.

Press MANUAL and set timer to 15 minutes.

The Pressure Pot will start building pressure; allow the mixture to cook for the set time.

When the timer reads zero, press QPR for quick pressure release.

Open the lid and take out the prepared recipe.

Serve warm.

Nutrition (per serving)

Calories 314,

Fat 19 g,

Carbs 14.5 g,

Protein 17 g,

Sodium 745 mg

Chickpea Spiced Chicken

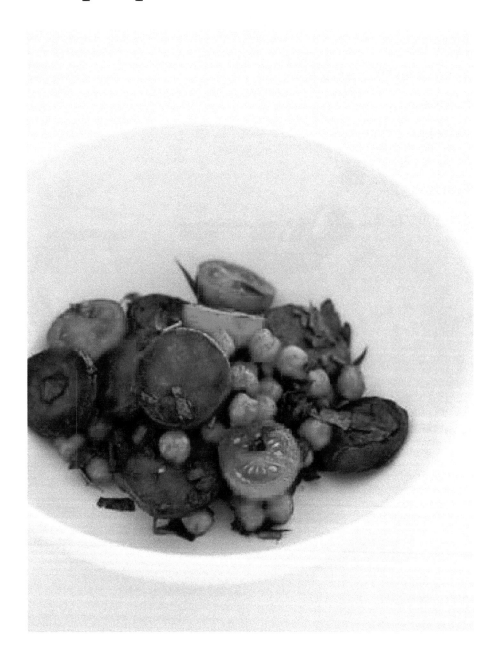

Difficulty Level: 2/5

Preparation time 10 minutes

Cooking time 15 minutes

Servings: 4

Ingredients

2 red peppers, cut into chunks

1 large onion

1 (15-ounce) can chickpeas

4 cloves garlic

2 roma tomatoes, cut into chunks

1 tablespoon olive oil

1–2 pounds boneless chicken thighs, trimmed and cut into large chunks

1 teaspoon cumin

½ teaspoon coriander powder

1 teaspoon salt

½ teaspoon pepper

1 teaspoon dried parsley

½ teaspoon red pepper flakes

1 cup tomato sauce

Directions

Open the top lid of your Pressure Pot and press SAUTÉ.

Add the olive oil to the pot and heat it.

Add the onions and garlic and stir-cook for 4–5 minutes until soft and translucent.

Add chicken chunks; stir-cook for 4–5 minutes on each side to evenly brown.

Add the remaining ingredients and stir gently.

Close the lid and make sure that the valve is sealed properly.

Press MANUAL and set timer to 10 minutes.

The Pressure Pot will start building pressure; allow the mixture to cook for the set time.

When the timer reads zero, press QPR for quick pressure release.

Open the lid and take out the prepared recipe.

Serve warm with grilled pita (optional).

Nutrition (per serving)

Calories 371,

Fat 15 g,

Carbs 26.5 g,

Protein 33 g,

Sodium 1279 mg

Vegetable Rice Chicken

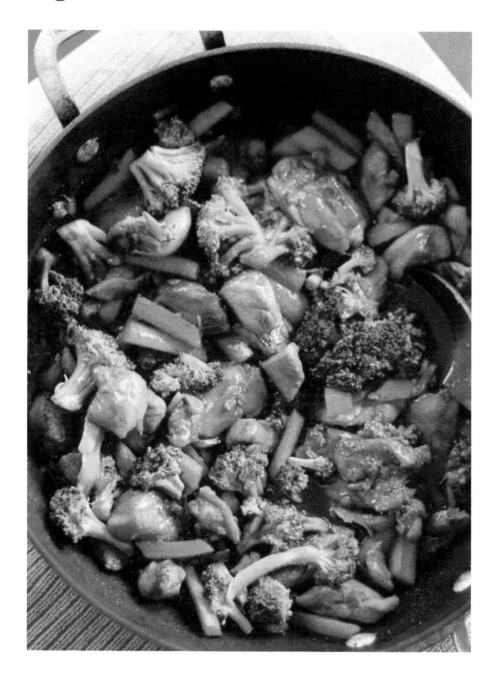

Difficulty Level: 2/5

Preparation time 10 minutes

Cooking time 4 minutes

Servings: 4

Ingredients

1 medium red onion, diced

4 cloves garlic, minced

2 tablespoons olive oil

3 chicken breasts, diced

3 tablespoons lemon juice

1½ cups chicken broth

1 each red and yellow bell pepper, chopped

1 zucchini, sliced

1 cup dry white rice

¼ cup parsley, finely chopped

1 tablespoon oregano

½ teaspoon each salt and pepper

¼ cup feta cheese, crumbled (optional)

Directions

Open the top lid of your Pressure Pot.

Add the olive oil, garlic, onions, chicken, lemon juice, oregano, salt and pepper; stir to combine with a wooden spatula.

Add the broth and rice; stir again.

Close the lid and make sure that the valve is sealed properly.

Press MANUAL and set timer to 4 minutes.

The Pressure Pot will start building pressure; allow the mixture to cook for the set time.

When the timer reads zero, press QPR for quick pressure release.

Open the lid and stir in the bell peppers, zucchini and parsley. Close the lid and allow to settle for 5–10 minutes.

Serve warm with the feta cheese on top (optional).

Nutrition (per serving)

Calories 293,

Fat 11 g,

Carbs 33.5 g,

Protein 16 g,

Sodium 951 mg

Chicken Shawarma

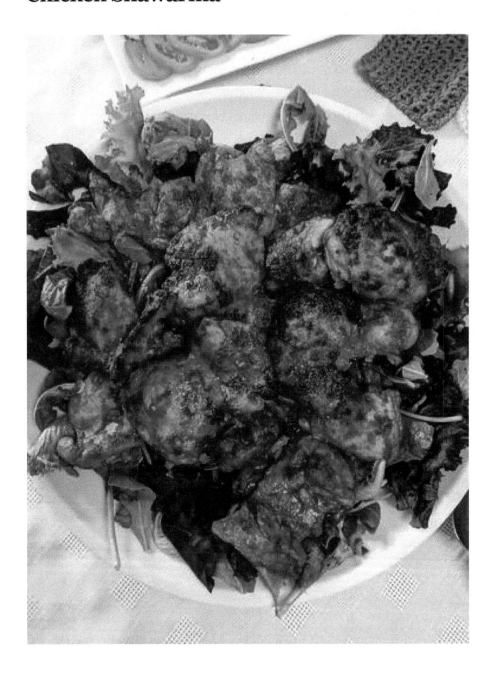

Difficulty Level: 2/5

Preparation time: 10 minutes

Cooking time: 15 minutes

Servings: 2-4

Ingredients

1–1½ pounds boneless skinless chicken thighs, cut into strips

1–1½ pounds boneless skinless chicken breasts, cut into strips

½ teaspoon turmeric

1 teaspoon ground cumin

1 teaspoon paprika

¼ teaspoon granulated garlic

⅛ teaspoon ground cinnamon

¼ teaspoon ground allspice

¼ teaspoon chili powder

Salt and pepper to taste

1 cup chicken broth or stock

Directions

Combine the spices in a mixing bowl. Add the strips and coat well. Season to taste with salt and pepper.

Open the top lid of your Pressure Pot.

Add the broth and chicken strips; stir to combine with a wooden spatula.

Close the lid and make sure that the valve is sealed properly.

Press MANUAL and set timer to 15 minutes.

The Pressure Pot will start building pressure; allow the mixture to cook for the set time.

When the timer reads zero, press QPR for quick pressure release.

Open the lid and take out the prepared recipe.

Serve warm with cooked veggies of your choice (optional).

Nutrition (per serving)

Calories 273,

Fat 9 g,

Carbs 12.5 g,

Protein 39.5 g,

Sodium 1149 mg

Caprese Chicken Dinner

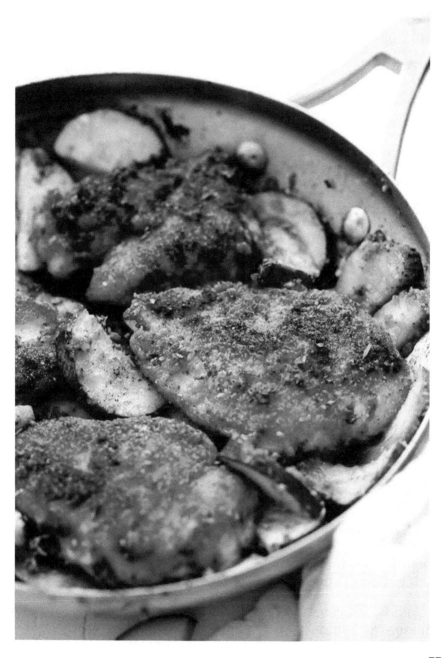

Difficulty Level: 2/5

Preparation time: 10 minutes

Cooking time 20 minutes

Servings: 6

Ingredients

¼ cup maple syrup or honey

¼ cup chicken stock or water

¼ cup balsamic vinegar

1½ pounds boneless skinless chicken thighs, fat trimmed

8 slices mozzarella cheese

3 cups cherry tomatoes

½ cup basil leaves, torn

Directions

Open the top lid of your Pressure Pot.

Add the stock, balsamic vinegar and maple syrup; stir to combine with a wooden spatula.

Add the chicken thighs and combine well.

Close the lid and make sure that the valve is sealed properly.

Press MANUAL and set timer to 10 minutes.

The Pressure Pot will start building pressure; allow the mixture to cook for the set time.

When the timer reads zero, press QPR for quick pressure release.

Open the lid, remove the chicken thighs, and place them on a baking sheet. Top each thigh with a cheese slice.

Press SAUTÉ; cook the sauce mixture for 4–5 minutes. Add the tomatoes and simmer for 1–2 minutes. Mix in the basil.

Add the baking sheet to a broiler and heat until the cheese melts. Serve warm with the sauce drizzled on top.

Nutrition (per serving)

Calories 311,

Fat 13 g,

Carbs 15 g,

Protein 31 g,

Sodium 364 mg

Pork Loin with Peach Sauce

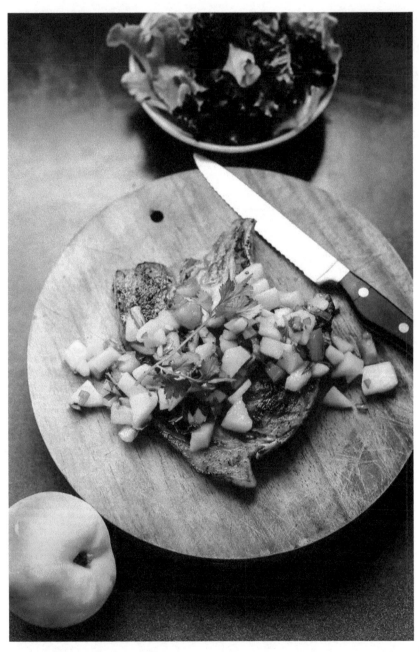

Difficulty Level: 2/5

Preparation time: 10 minutes

Cooking time 10 minutes

Servings: 4

Ingredients

1 (15-ounce) can peaches, diced (liquid reserved)

¼ cup beef stock

1 pound pork loin, cut into chunks

2 tablespoons white wine

2 tablespoons sweet chili sauce

2 tablespoons soy sauce

2 tablespoons honey

¼ cup water combined with 2 tablespoons cornstarch

Directions

Open the top lid of your Pressure Pot.

Add the wine, soy sauce, beef stock, peach can liquid and chili sauce; stir to combine with a wooden spatula.

Add the pork and stir again.

Close the lid and make sure that the valve is sealed properly.

Press MANUAL and set timer to 5 minutes.

The Pressure Pot will start building pressure; allow the mixture to cook for the set time.

When the timer reads zero, press NPR for natural pressure release. It will take 8–10 minutes to release the pressure.

Open the lid and mix in the cornstarch mixture.

Press SAUTÉ; cook for 4–5 minutes. Mix in the peach pieces.

Serve warm.

Nutrition (per serving)

Calories 277,

fat 4.5 g,

carbs 28 g,

protein 24 g,

sodium 1133 mg

Mushroom Tomato Beef

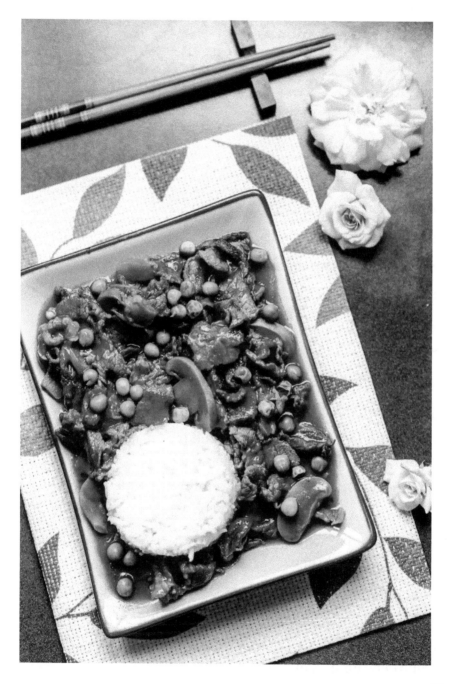

Difficulty Level: 2/5

Preparation time: 10 minutes

Cooking time 18 minutes

Servings: 4

Ingredients

1 pound beef steaks

1 bay leaf

1 tablespoon dried thyme

6 ounces cherry tomatoes

1 pound button mushrooms, thinly chopped

2 tablespoons extra-virgin olive oil or avocado oil

½ teaspoon pepper

1 teaspoon salt

Directions

Rub the steaks with salt, pepper and thyme.

Open the top lid of your Pressure Pot.

Add the bay leaf, 3 cups of water, and the steaks; stir to combine with a wooden spatula.

Close the lid and make sure that the valve is sealed properly.

Press MANUAL and set timer to 13 minutes.

The Pressure Pot will start building pressure; allow the mixture to cook for the set time.

When the timer reads zero, press QPR for quick pressure release.

Open the lid and take out the prepared recipe.

Add the olive oil to the pot and SAUTÉ the tomatoes and mushrooms for 4–5 minutes.

Add the steak and stir-cook to evenly brown. Serve warm.

Nutrition (per serving)

Calories 384,

Fat 21 g,

Carbs 11 g,

Protein 23.5 g,

Sodium 664 mg

Black Olive Sea Bass
Difficulty Level: 2/5

Preparation time: 10 minutes

Cooking time 4 minutes

Servings: 4

Ingredients

12 cherry tomatoes

12 black olives

2 tablespoons marinated baby capers

¼ cup water

4 frozen sea bass or other white fish fillets, halved

½ teaspoon salt

Pinch of chili flakes

⅓ cup roasted red peppers, sliced

2 tablespoons olive oil

Fresh parsley or basil, chopped, to serve

Directions

Open the top lid of your Pressure Pot.

Add the water and frozen fish. Add the remaining ingredients and top with the olive oil, sea salt and chili flakes.

Close the lid and make sure that the valve is sealed properly.

Press MANUAL and set timer to 4 minutes.

The Pressure Pot will start building pressure; allow the mixture to cook for the set time.

When the timer reads zero, press NPR for natural pressure release. It will take 8–10 minutes to release the pressure.

Open the lid and take out the prepared recipe.

Serve warm with basil or parsley on top.

Note: If using fresh fish, set timer to 5 minutes at LOW pressure.

Nutrition (per serving)

Calories 224,

Fat 12.5 g,

Carbs 4.5 g,

Protein 24 g,

Sodium 824 mg

Broccoli Soy Salmon

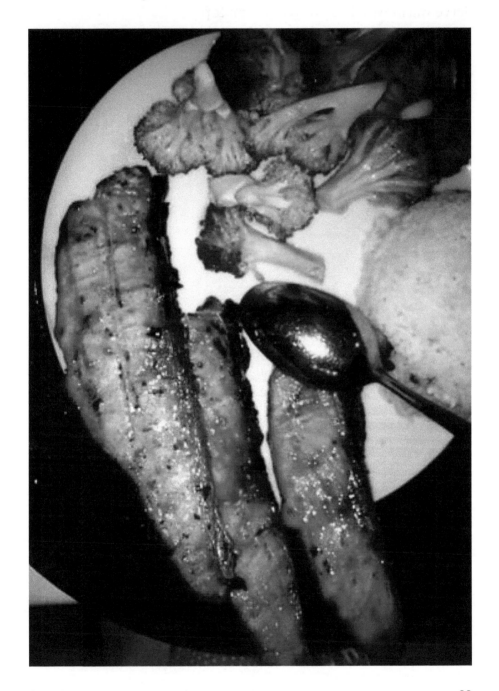

Difficulty Level: 2/5

Preparation time: 10 minutes

Cooking time 2 minutes

Servings: 4

Ingredients

1 pound Alaskan salmon, cut into four 4-ounce fillets

Salt and pepper to taste

Dressing:

1 pound broccoli, cut into florets

2 tablespoons raw apple cider vinegar

6 tablespoons extra-virgin olive oil

2 tablespoons soy sauce or tamari

3 tablespoons maple syrup

1 teaspoon toasted sesame oil

1 tablespoon fresh ginger, minced

1 clove garlic

Sesame seeds and chopped green onions for garnish

Directions

Blend the sesame oil, olive oil, ginger, garlic, soy sauce, vinegar and maple syrup in a blender. Set aside.

Open the top lid of your Pressure Pot.

Add 1 cup of water to the cooking pot; arrange the trivet/steamer basket.

Place the salmon fillets skin side down over the steamer basket/trivet. Season with salt and pepper.

Close the lid and make sure that the valve is sealed properly.

Press MANUAL and set timer to 1 minute.

The Pressure Pot will start building pressure; allow the mixture to cook for the set time.

When the timer reads zero, press QPR for quick pressure release.

Open the lid and place the broccoli over the salmon.

Close the lid and make sure that the valve is sealed properly.

Press MANUAL and set timer to 1 minute.

The Pressure Pot will start building pressure; allow the mixture to cook for the set time.

When the timer reads zero, press QPR for quick pressure release.

Open the lid and serve warm with the dressing, green onions and sesame seeds on top.

Nutrition (per serving)

Calories 395,

Fat 26 g,

Carbs 14 g,

Protein 27 g,

Sodium 654 mg

Shrimp Fennel Pasta

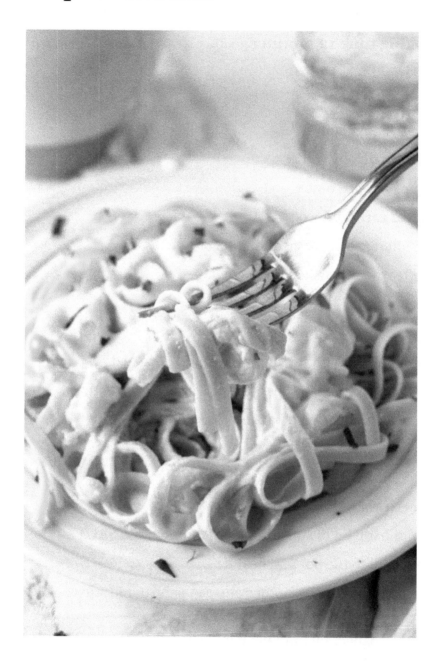

Difficulty Level: 2/5

Preparation time: 10 minutes

Cooking time 12 minutes

Servings: 6

Ingredients

1 small fennel bulb

1 tablespoon olive oil

½ cup chopped onion

6 cloves garlic, minced

1 (28-ounce) can crushed tomatoes

½–1 teaspoon crushed red pepper

2¾ cups water

⅓ cup cognac or brandy

1 pound raw jumbo shrimp, peeled and deveined

1 pound dried whole wheat trottole pasta or corkscrews

2 tablespoons chopped parsley

Salt and pepper to taste

3 tablespoons heavy cream

Directions

Open the top lid of your Pressure Pot and press SAUTÉ.

Add the oil to the pot and heat it.

Add the fennel, garlic, onions and red pepper and stir-cook for 3–5 minutes to soften.

Add the cognac, salt and pepper, tomatoes, water and pasta. Stir the mixture.

Close the lid and make sure that the valve is sealed properly.

Press MANUAL and set timer to 4 minutes.

The Pressure Pot will start building pressure; allow the mixture to cook for the set time.

When the timer reads zero, press QPR for quick pressure release.

Open the lid and mix in the cream, shrimp and parsley.

Press SAUTÉ; cook the mixture for 2–3 minutes.

Serve warm.

Nutrition (per serving)

Calories 491,

fat 7 g,

carbs 61 g,

protein 28 g,

sodium 797 mg

Fish with Farro & Green Beans
Difficulty Level: 2/5

Preparation time: 10 minutes

Cooking time 12 minutes

Servings: 4

Ingredients

4 skinless trout fillets

½ pound green beans

1 cup farro

2 cups water

1 tablespoon olive oil

1 teaspoon salt (divided)

1 teaspoon pepper (divided)

½ tablespoon sugar

¼ cup melted butter

½ teaspoon dried rosemary

2 cloves garlic, minced

½ teaspoon dried thyme

½ tablespoon lemon juice

Directions

In a mixing bowl, combine the green beans, olive oil, ½ teaspoon of the pepper, and ½ teaspoon of the salt.

In another bowl, combine the remaining salt and pepper with the butter, sugar, garlic, lemon juice and rosemary. Add the fish and coat well.

Open the top lid of your Pressure Pot.

Add the water and farro; season with some salt.

Arrange the trivet/steamer basket. Place the trout fillets and green beans over it.

Close the lid and make sure that the valve is sealed properly.

Press MANUAL and set timer to 12 minutes.

The Pressure Pot will start building pressure; allow the mixture to cook for the set time.

When the timer reads zero, press QPR for quick pressure release.

Open the lid and take out the prepared recipe. Serve warm.

Nutrition (per serving)

Calories 331,

Fat 16.5 g,

Carbs 36 g,

Protein 12 g,

Sodium 602 mg

Spinach Mackerel
Difficulty Level: 2/5

Preparation time: 10 minutes

Cooking time 12 minutes

Serves 4

Ingredients

5 potatoes, peeled and chopped

¼ cup olive oil

4 mackerels, skin on

1 pound spinach, torn

1 teaspoon dried rosemary, chopped

2 cloves garlic, crushed

1 lemon, juiced

2 sprigs mint leaves, chopped

Salt to taste

Directions

Open the top lid of your Pressure Pot and press SAUTÉ.

Add the olive oil to the pot and heat it.

Add the garlic and rosemary; stir-cook for 1–2 minutes until fragrant.

Add the spinach and a pinch of salt and cook for 4–5 minutes, until the spinach wilts. Remove the spinach and set aside.

Add the potatoes and fish and top with the sea salt and lemon juice.

Add 1 cup of water.

Close the lid and make sure that the valve is sealed properly.

Press STEAM and set timer to 7 minutes.

The Pressure Pot will start building pressure; allow the mixture to cook for the set time.

When the timer reads zero, press QPR for quick pressure release.

Open the lid and take out the prepared recipe. Serve the fish warm with the spinach on top.

Nutrition (per serving)

Calories 289,

Fat 12 g,

Carbs 13.5 g,

Protein 21 g,

Sodium 733 mg

Pressure Pot Beef Gyros

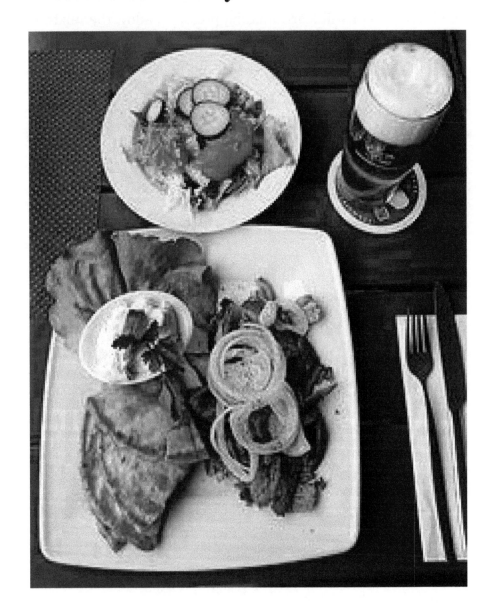

Difficulty Level: 2/5

Preparation time: *10 minutes*

Cooking time: 15 minutes

Servings: 6

Ingredients:

2 pounds beef roast, thinly sliced

1 tablespoon dried parsley

1 teaspoon salt

3 cloves minced garlic

1 teaspoon black pepper

1 sliced red onion

4 tablespoons oil of choice

1 teaspoon olive oil

½ cup vegetable broth

1 tablespoon lemon juice

For the Tzatziki sauce:

1 cup plain yogurt

1 clove minced garlic

2 tablespoon fresh dill

½ cup cucumber, peeled, seeded, and chopped finely

Directions:

Turn on Pressure Pot and then add oil to the bottom.

Add meat, seasonings, garlic, and onion to sear and soften the onions.

Pour the lemon juice and broth over meat, and then stir it, lock lid into place, and then use meat/stew and cook it for 9 minutes.

Let it natural release pressure for 3 minutes before quickly released.

Mix the Tzatziki sauce and if you want vegetable toppings or apple cider vinegar over this, you can.

You can also put lettuce at the bottom of naan or pita bread before adding meat and toppings.

Nutrition:

Calories: 395,

Fat: 27g

Carbs: 4gNet

Carbs: 4g

Protein: 32g

Fiber: 0g.

Sodium 38%

Pressure Pot Lasagna Hamburger Helper

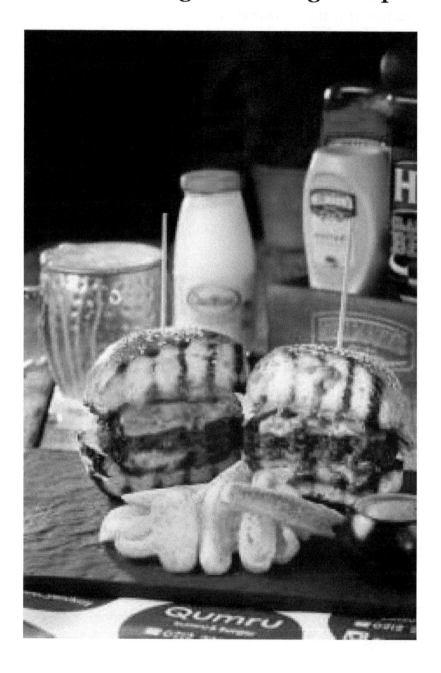

Difficulty Level: 2/5

Preparation time: *2 minutes*

Cooking time: 5 minutes

Serves: 4

Ingredients:

1 box 16 oz, pasta

8 oz. Ricotta cheese

½ pound ground beef

1 jar pasta sauce

8 oz. Mozzarella cheese

½ pound ground sausage

4 cups water

Directions:

Put pot in sauté mood and cook meat till brown and crumbled.

Add in rest of ingredients, turn it on high pressure for five minutes.

Quick release it, and then put in half the cheese and half the mozzarella, and then put into a baking pan with more mozzarella. You can cook it for another 2-3 minutes till cheese melts.

Nutrition:

Calories: 537

Fat: 33g

Carbs: 25 g

Protein: 34g

Fiber: 4g

Sodium 36%

Healthy Pressure Pot Mediterranean Chicken

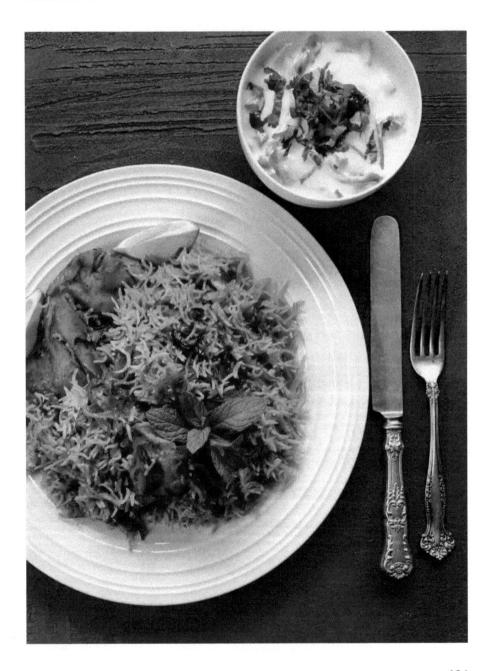

Difficulty Level: 2/5

Preparation time: 5 minutes

Cooking time: 20 minutes

Servings: 4

Ingredients:

4 chicken breasts, skinless and boneless

1 can tomatoes with no salt, diced

½ onion, diced

2 tablespoons garlic, minced

25 kalamata or black olives, pitted

2 tablespoons extra virgin olive oil

2 tablespoons Greek seasoning

fresh oregano sprigs for garnish

Directions:

Cut each chicken breast into 4-5 large pieces.

Turn Pressure Pot to the sauté setting.

Add the olive oil, onion, and garlic to the pot. Cook for 3-4 minutes.

Sprinkle Greek seasoning on both sides of chicken pieces.

Take ½ of chicken breasts and place them in the Pressure Pot. Brown on both sides, which will take about 3 minutes. Remove this first batch of chicken and add in the second. Once this chicken is done, remove from the pot.

Add the tomatoes, olives and dried oregano.

Nestle the chicken breasts into olive oil mixture.

Set the Pressure Pot to Manual high for 15 minutes.

Allow to self-release for 10 minutes and then pressure release until all of the steam is gone.

Serve this chicken over your favorite rice.

Nutrition: (Per serving)

Calories: 228

Protein: 11.1 grams

Total Fat: 10.7 grams

Carbohydrates: 25 grams

Lightning Source UK Ltd.
Milton Keynes UK
UKHW020659310521
384668UK00001B/31